Natural Massage Oil Recipes

By

Gene Ashburner

ISBN-13:978-1505898286
ISBN-10:1505898285

Content

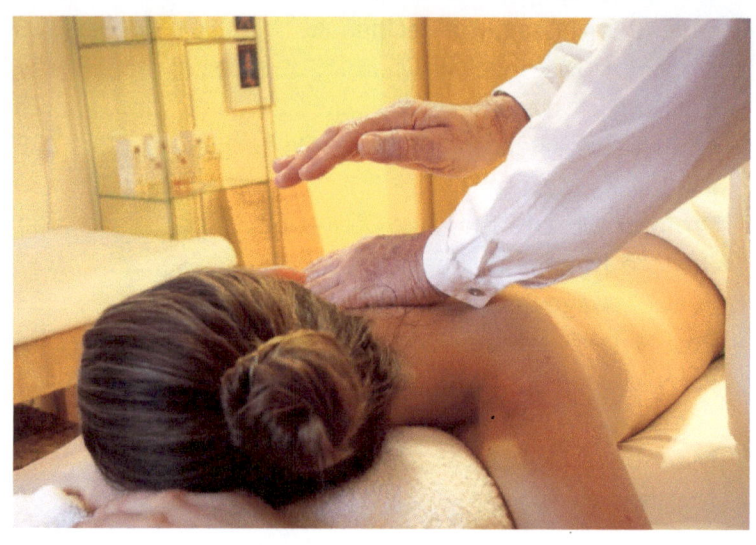

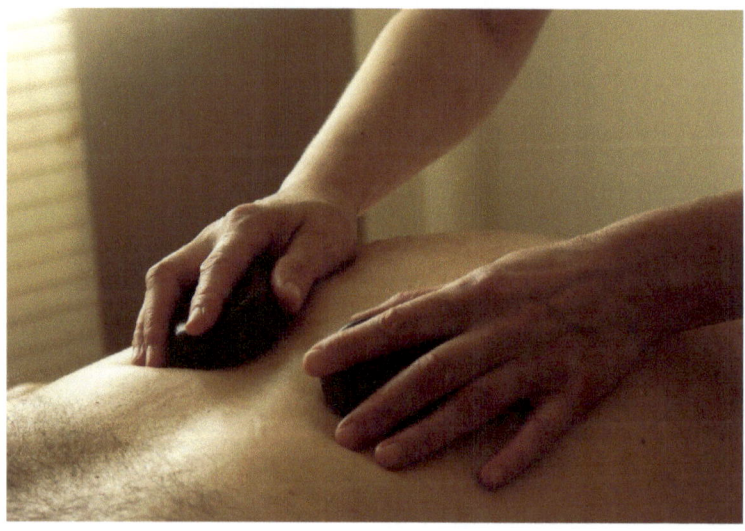

Massage Is Said To Be Therapeutic

It is the science of healing that involves the human touch. For several decades now, people have been making use of this option to treat their physical and emotional problems. One of the most popular types is the Thai massage therapy.

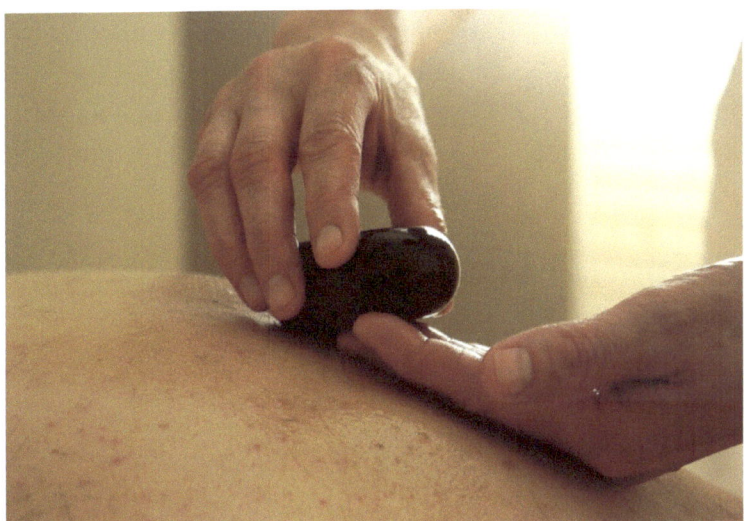

Types Of Massage

1. Thai Massage

Thai massage is one of the types that have been practiced for a long time. Its existence can be traced to more than a thousand years now. The therapy itself forms part of the well-known area of Thai medicine. It comprises of manipulation, medicinal treatment, ritual, and diet.

It is rooted from the belief that each and every disease is caused by a particular imbalance in the energy system within the body. It is geared at the promotion of balance which hence aids in the complete healing and rejuvenation of an individual.

2. Sports Massage

This treatment incorporates several massage techniques which is great for athletes.

- It keeps the body flexible

- Increases performance

- Assists in rehabilitation from an injury

3. Swedish Massage

This is probably the most common form of massage in the US.

Its main goal is relaxation and improved circulation. The therapist applies oil to the skin and uses flowing strokes and kneading movements to relieve tension from the muscles.

4. Deep Tissue Massage

This type of massage is more vigorous and uses various styles to loosen the muscles.

It helps break patterns of:

- Tension

- Relieves chronic pain

- Inflammation-related pain such as tendonitis

- Improves range of motion

5. Craniosacral Therapy

This therapy involves the Craniosacral system which extends from the skull to the bottom of the spine and consists of the brain, spinal cord, cerebrospinal fluid and surrounding membranes.

This can help treat such conditions as:

- Headaches

- Eye problems

- Ear problems

- Whiplash

- Back pain

6. Pregnancy Massage

This massage focuses on a pregnant woman's needs including swollen hands and feet, stress on weight-bearing joints, exhaustion and lower back pain. And of course the practitioner positions you to accommodate your baby bump.

7. Tantric Massage

They are recognized for their aphrodisiac, numbing, calming, and drowsy effects.

For tantric massage, the following oils are advisable

- Ginger

- Black Pepper

- Geranium

- Fennel

- Pine

- Juniper

- Rosemary

- Sandalwood

Use Of Massage Oils

By applying a massage oil or ointment at the area you work at, you ease the massage work and increase the effects of the massage. Your fingers glide more easily upon the skin covering the area. The blood supply of the skin and muscles will be stimulated. You get a sensual and exciting scent on the area and in the air. Ingredients in the oil will ameliorate muscular ache and pain. According to the composition of the massage oil, there will be different stimulating effects upon the muscles, for example faster regeneration of tired or hurt muscle tissue.

Commonly Used Carrier Oils

Carrier oils provide much needed lubrication allowing hands to move freely over the skin, helping with the absorption of essential oils into the body. Carrier oils are light, non sticky and effectively penetrate the skin. They should be 100% pure, unrefined and cold pressed.

Dilution:

1 drop of essential oil = 1 tsp of carrier oil for 1% dilution.

2 drops essential oil to 1 tsp of carrier oil = 2% dilution and so on.

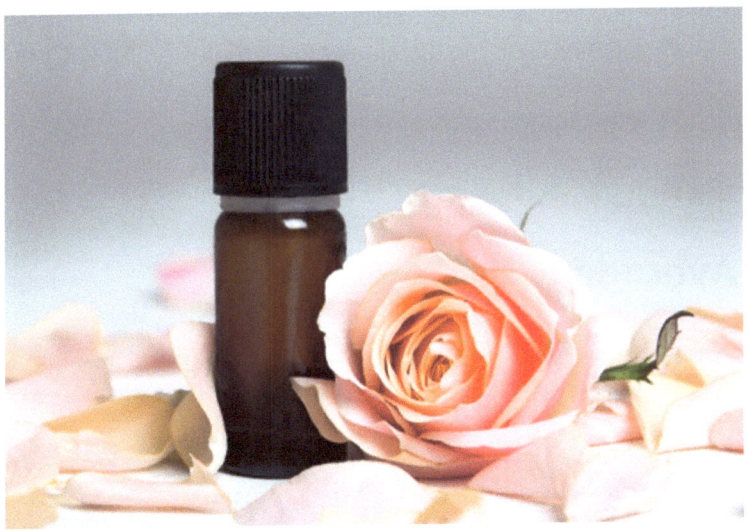

Apricot Kernel Oil

Extracted from the kernel of the apricot fruit, it is pale yellow in colour. This oil is light and easily absorbed.

Contains:

- Vitamins A and B help in healing and rejuvenating skin cells.

- Contains vitamin E.

Used For:

- Good for all skin types especially for sensitive, inflamed and dry skin.

- Excellent oil for facial area.

- It leaves skin soft and supple.

- It moisturizes both the body and face.

Avocado Oil

Refined avocado oil is preferred as it lacks odor.

Contains:

- It is rich in lecithin, vitamins, A, D, and E.

- It delays anti aging as it is rich in essential fatty acids.

Used For:

- Used for intensive facial treatment for mature skin.

- Easily penetrates the skin, acts as sunscreen and helps in cell regeneration.

Peanut Oil

Peanut oil has an extremely light aroma with a faintly nutty quality. Its texture is thick and leaves a very oily film on the skin and its color is almost clear.

Used For:

- Use caution with peanut oil as it should not be used on anyone who has an allergy to peanuts.

- Its oily texture can help with arthritis.

Wheat Germ Oil

Contains:

- Highly nourishing oil with vitamin E.

Used For:

- Perfect oil for dry, mature and lifeless skin.

Grape Seed Oil

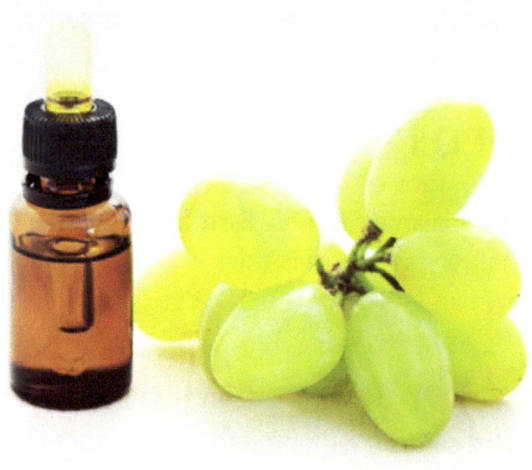

Odorless unlike most oils, it is light and good for skin not absorbing other oils. No greasy feeling after application.

Contains:

- Grape seed oil is safe to use because of its non-allergenic components.

Used For:

- Slightly astringent, it tightens, tones the skin and alleviates acne.

- It is an ideal carrier for body massage.

Jojoba Oil

It is one of the best oils for hair and skin.

Good for all skin types, but clogs pores sometimes.

It promotes a healthy, glowing complexion.

Penetrates the skin quickly, excellent for skin nourishment.

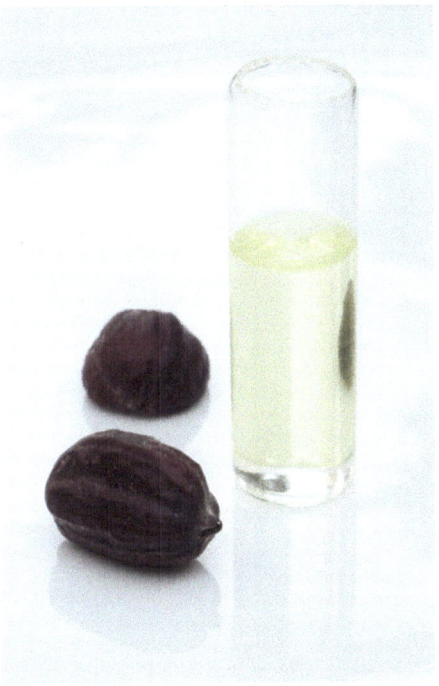

Used For:

■ Controls acne, oily skin or scalp as excess sebum dissolves in jojoba.

- Good base oil for treating rheumatism and arthritis.

- It heals inflamed skin, psoriasis, eczema, or any sort of dermatitis.

Rosehip Oil

It is called the queen of carrier oil. Cold pressed from the seeds of rose hips, it pale yellow light texture.

It is wonderful carrier oil for skin care.

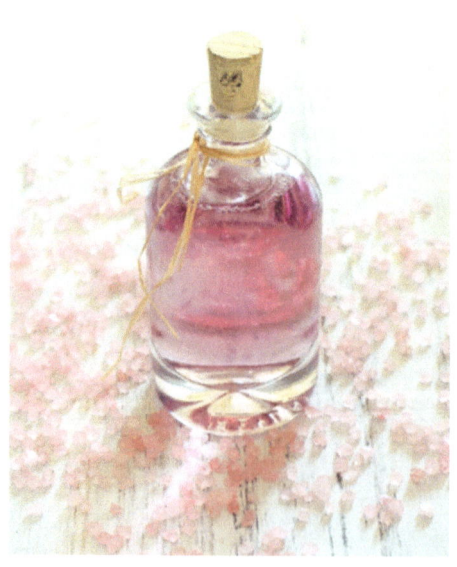

Used For:

- Good oil for cosmetic, cell regeneration prevents premature skin aging and softens wrinkles.

- Good for eczema, psoriasis, PMS and menopause.

- When combined with calendula oil, it treats stretch marks, burns or scars.

Sweet Almond Oil

Popular carrier oil in body massage. Lubricates and moisturizes the skin. Quickly absorbs into the skin, leaving your skin to feel soft and non greasy.

Contains:

- Rich in proteins and vitamin D.

Used For:

- Provides relief from itching, soreness, dryness, inflammation.

- Good for all skin types, especially eczema.

Calendula Oil

Infusion of marigold flowers, renowned for its soothing properties.

Used For:

- Balances excessively oily skin.

- Can be used alone or blended with almond or grape seed oil for body massage.

Evening Primrose Oil

Used For:

- Perfect skincare oil for moisturizing, softening and soothing to dry and irritated skin.

Sunflower Oil

Has good softening and moisturizing properties.

Used For:

- Used for facial treatments and body massage.

St. John Wort Oil

Infusions from the Hypericum bush.

Used For:

- It is excellent for all types of sensitive, red and sore skin.

Coconut Oil

Light, easily absorbable into the skin giving smooth satin effect.

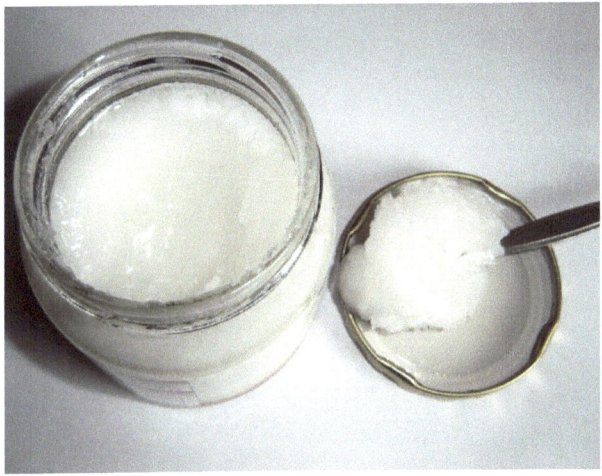

Used For:

- Perfect moisturizer for body and hands.

- Moisturizes and conditions brittle, dull or dry hair.

Common Herbs That Are Used In Essential Oils

Lavender

Lavender helps relieve tired muscles and can actually reduce muscle spasms.

Bergamot

Bergamot is very uplifting

Tea Tree

Tea tree oil is an herb that is often used in topical mixtures to help fight bacterial infections.

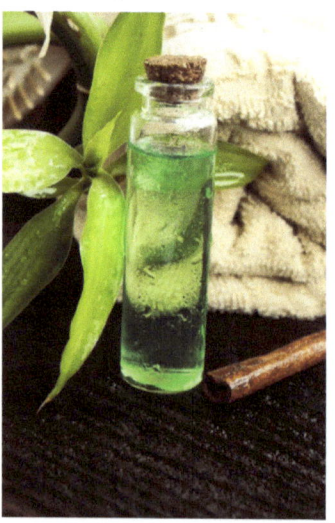

Neroli

Neroli is often used to help control the signs of stress and anxiety.

Melissa

Melissa is known for its antiseptic properties when used on the skin.

Frankincense

It is used to help restore confidence and calm.

Juniper

Juniper is used to clear and stimulate the mind.

Grape seed

Slightly astringent, it tightens, tones the skin and alleviates acne. It is an ideal carrier for body massage.

Jasmine oil

It helps lift your mood and ease stress.

Sweet almond

Gives relief from itching, soreness, dryness, inflammation.

Bay oil

Bay oil can be used in the treatment of rheumatism, neuralgia, muscular pain, circulation problems, colds, flu, dental infection, hair growth, general health of the scalp, diarrhea and skin infections.

Castor oil

Improves lymphatic flow.

Lime oil

Uplifting and refreshing.

Rosemary oil

Effective for mental fatigue, circulation problems, pain relief for the muscular system, decongests the respiratory tract and is a skin and hair booster.

Sandalwood

Relaxes nerves, muscles and blood vessels and hence ends spasm or contraction.

Massaging Oil Recipes

Indulging Massage Oil Recipe

Ingredients

40 ml grape seed oil (tightens and tones the skin, ideal carrier for body massage)

6 drops of jasmine oil (helps lift mood and ease stress)

2 drops tea tree oil (helps fight bacterial infections)

2 drops Neroli oil (helps control the signs of stress and anxiety)

Method

Combine all the ingredients together and blend well.

Before application warm the oil.

Lavender Massage Oil Recipe

Ingredients

> 12 drops lavender oil (relieves tired muscles)
>
> 37,5 ml carrier oil of choice (see section on carrier oils)

Method

Combine all the ingredients together and blend well.

Before application warm the oil.

Masculine Massage Oil

Ingredients

- 62,5 ml grape seed oil (tightens and tones the skin, ideal carrier for body massage)
- 31 ml castor oil (improves lymphatic flow)
- 31 ml sweet almond oil (relief from itching, soreness, dryness, inflammation)
- 6 drops sandalwood oil (relaxes nerves, muscles and blood vessels)
- 4 drops bay oil (helps with rheumatism, neuralgia and muscular pain)
- 3 drops bergamot oil (is very uplifting)
- 2 drops lime oil (uplifting and refreshing)

Method

Combine all the ingredients together and blend well.

Before application warm the oil.

Relaxing Massage Recipe

Ingredients

50 ml carrier oil of choice (see section on carrier oils)

10 drops lavender oil (relieves tired muscles)

10 drops rosemary oil (for mental fatigue, circulation, pain relief for the muscular system and skin booster)

10 drops bergamot oil (is very uplifting)

Method

Combine all the ingredients together and blend well.

Before application warm the oil.

Frankincense Relaxing Massage Oil Recipe

Ingredients

   4 drops frankincense (it is used to help restore confidence and calm)

   50 ml carrier oil of choice (see section on carrier oils)

Method

Combine all the ingredients together and blend well.

Before application warm the oil.

Petit grain Massage Oil Recipe

Ingredients

    4 drops petit grain oil (calm the nervous system)

    50 ml carrier oil of choice (see section on carrier oils)

Method

Combine all the ingredients together and blend well.

Before application warm the oil.

Promote Dreams Massage Oil Recipe

Ingredients

50 ml grape seed oil (tightens and tones the skin, ideal carrier for body massage)

6 drops chamomile oil (enhances overall feelings of calm and relaxation)

4 drops jasmine oil (helps lift mood and ease stress)

2 drops rose oil (soothing effect)

1 drop lavender oil (relieves tired muscles)

Method

Combine all the ingredients together and blend well.

Before application warm the oil.

Restore The Beauty Recipe

This massage oil is to help keep mature skin supple and smooth

Ingredients

- 25 ml carrier oil of choice (see section on carrier oils)
- 25 ml rosehip seed oil (prevents premature skin aging)
- 10 drops palm rose oil (moisturizes and hydrate all skin types)
- 10 drops lavender oil (relieves tired muscles)
- 10 drops patchouli oil (has anti aging properties)

Method

Combine all the ingredients together and blend well.

Before application warm the oil.

Feet Massage Recipe

Ingredients

50 ml carrier oil of choice (see section on carrier oils)

10 drops spearmint oil (helps with fatigue and stress)

5 drops wintergreen oil (for joints and muscles)

5 drops rosemary oil (for circulation)

Method

Combine all the ingredients together and blend well.

Before application warm the oil.

Post Natal Depression Massage Recipe

Ingredients

> 8 drops geranium oil (helps with stress, anxiety and depression)
>
> 10 drops grapefruit (lymph drainage)
>
> 6 drops mandarin oil (soothing, rejuvenating and refreshing)

Method

Combine all the ingredients together and blend well.

Before application warm the oil.

Baby Massage Recipe

Ingredients

25 ml sweet almond oil (lubricates and moisturizes the skin)

5 drops lavender essential oil (promotes restful sleep)

Method

Combine all the ingredients together and blend well.

Before application warm the oil.

For Couples Only Massage Oil Recipe

Ingredients

25 ml carrier oil of choice (see section on carrier oils)

25 ml rosehip seed oil (prevents premature skin aging)

10 drops patchouli oil (has anti aging properties)

10 drops lemongrass oil (soothing and calming effect)

10 drops vanilla oil (stimulates secretion of testosterone and estrogen which help bring about normal sexual behavior and promotes arousal)

Method

Combine all the ingredients together and blend well.

Before application warm the oil.

Menopausal Sweats Massage Recipe

Ingredients

10 drops grapefruit oil (lymph drainage)

10 drops lime oil (uplifting and refreshing)

7 drops sage oil (strengthen the senses)

3 drops thyme oil (circulatory system, heart, digestive system, nervous system, muscles and skin, fortify them and boosts immunity)

25 ml carrier oil choice (see section on carrier oils)

Method

Combine all the ingredients together and blend well.

Before application warm the oil.

Massage Oil For PMS

Ingredients

> 5 drops carrot seed oil (rejuvenate the energy of the solar plexus)
>
> 10 drops clary sage oil (uterine tonic)
>
> 10 drops fennel oil (properties of fennel oil are emenagogue, carminative, depurative, diuretic, laxative and stimulant)
>
> 20 drops lavender oil - (relieves tired muscles)
>
> 30 drops marjoram oil (soothing, warming and fortifying, may induce menstruation for some where their cycle has been inconsistent)
>
> 5 drops mugwort oil (emenagogue - the blocked menstruations can be restarted)
>
> 20 drops rosewood oil (stimulates feelings, secretions of hormones)
>
> 125 ml carrier oil of choice (see section on carrier oils)

Method

Combine all the ingredients together and blend well.

Before application warm the oil.

www.ingramcontent.com/pod-product-compliance
Lightning Source LLC
Chambersburg PA
CBHW050757290526
45792CB00008B/2221